FOREVER
FIT

Putting More Years in Your
Life and More Life in Your Years

FOREVER
FIT

Putting More Years in Your
Life and More Life in Your Years

Lisa Dumont

*BS Nutritional Sciences, ACE Certified Personal
Trainer, Functional Aging Specialist
Co-Authored by Dan Ritchie, PhD*

Published in partnership with the Functional Aging Institute

Published by Niche Pressworks
Book publishing for business builders.
nichepressworks.com

I wish to thank the following people for sharing their inspirational stories and helping me make this book a reality…..Guy Wood ,Corrie Haskell, Marsha Austin , Sue Higley, Wayne Wallace, Pam Baucom, Tress Zuverino, Pat and Barb Boylan , Becky Brown, Sandy Miller, MaryLou Smith, Brad and Bev Dunbar, Pam Prentiss and Doreen Woodward. You all are my heroes! I would also like to thank Craig Mellish- my photographer extraordinaire and The Dunbars for being my Cover models.

Table of Contents

Foreword

When you are pushing 80 will you have the ability and energy to travel halfway across the globe on an amazing adventure? Would you like to?

Bob came to me at the age of 79 so that I could train him for just that purpose. He had planned a bucket-list trip to hike the world's longest cave, the Son Doong cave, with his son-in-law and grandson.

Nestled in the lush jungle of Vietnam near the border of Laos, the cave is one of the world's most incredible and beautiful natural wonders containing a river, a lush forest, amazing rock formations, stalactites and more. Created millions of years ago by an underground river that eroded, the limestone cave is over 200m wide, 150m high and 9km long. Some of the caverns are so large that a small city could fit inside them. It takes explorers 6 hours of walking down a 10km narrow jungle path just to reach the mouth of the cave.

Visitors are warned that this is the easy part of the trip and that those who struggle getting to the cave will be turned away and not allowed to continue on the journey.

As you could expect, Bob was concerned that being the oldest one in the group would stop him from completing the trip. He didn't want to be the one to ruin the trip for his son-in-law and grandson after traveling so far and spending so much. Fortunately Bob had done a good job of staying in shape and you would never have guessed he was almost 80 years old. He certainly looked and moved like a man 15-20 years younger thanks to his regular exercise sessions that include treadmill walking and basic strength training.

We began his training using the techniques and strategies that you will find in this book. It became clear very early on that although his fitness program had paid off in many ways, he still had some areas of weakness that could put him at serious risk on his expedition. For example, Bob had a very difficult time moving his head in one direction while walking in another direction. He also struggled greatly performing certain crossover patterns with his feet. Think about how difficult it would be to hike on rocky, slippery terrain while also trying to visually take in all of the amazing beauty around you. What about when you step on a loose rock and have to quickly cross your feet over to keep your balance? Bob had a difficult time with both of these, which in my opinion, was a recipe for disaster.

Fortunately, Bob came to see me and I was able to apply our Functional Aging Training approach to greatly improve these and other critical areas in just a few short months. So how did his trip go? Funny you should ask. Bob survived the 6 hour walk down to the cave with flying colors...but his 40-something year old son-in-law, who hadn't trained like he should have, didn't fare so well. In fact, he struggled so much that they were NOT allowed to continue. It is sad really, but it highlights a very important fact - age should NEVER be a reason for slowing down and giving in. There are way too many great adventures still to come in life.

Over the years, we have seen thousands of middle-aged and older adults improve the quality of their life through transformational exercise programs that maximize physical function. This is why it is so important that you have this book in your hand right now, at this very moment in time. This is why we founded the Functional Aging Institute with the ultimate goal of impacting the lives of people just like you all around the globe!

Our goal is to help people realize that they can keep doing all the things they need to do, like to do and want to do for a very long time as long as they follow the exercise principles and strategies outlined in this book.

Whether it is playing with grandchildren, taking on a new career, climbing mountains, extending the years you get to play golf and tennis, or traveling around the world to exotic places...you can do it all into your 80's and 90's with greater ease and less pain.

This is where the Functional Aging Training model and the Functional Aging Institute comes in. We are currently on our way to our goal of having 10,000 certified Functional Aging Specialists all around the world who, over their careers, will guide 10-20 million people toward an entirely different aging trajectory. One that allows people like you to look forward to their next 20-30 years with joyful anticipation knowing that you are doing the best you possibly can to stay healthy and functional. By choosing to connect yourself with Lisa Dumont- Westminster Fit Body Bootcamp/ Fit Body Forever you're making a decision that will enrich your life, and the lives of all the people you love, for generations to come. We're grateful to contribute to that vision.

- Cody Sipe, PhD
Co-founder, Funtional Aging Institute

Preface

Is there anything you are NOT doing right now because your health and/or fitness is holding you back?

This book is for all of you out there who are willing to overcome your fears and concerns about aging and exercise by focusing on your goals and dreams, and in doing so, preserving your independence for as long as possible.

This is no ordinary book as it focuses on a segment of the population of which I am a proud member....... the Baby Boomers. I am excitedly entering into the 3rd phase of my life and I still have so much I want to do...... travel, ride horseback, give back to my community, play with my grandkids (should I ever have any), hike Macchu Picchu, **and MOST of all, helps others do all the things they want to do in life.**

If you are wondering how I can help you, then read on! I have had more than 30 years of experience coaching, motivating and educating thousands of clients about nutrition, exercise and personal development, I'm in the biz of "living the life of your dreams and my program is the vehicle to get there." I've come to believe that we all know we need to stay active, eat right and get proper rest so how come we all don't do it? It's about accountability sprinkled with a bit of motivation, having a plan and my secret weapon.........CARING. My programs are designed with YOU in mind. Once we get to know you better, we create a plan. For starters, each plan includes a safe and effective workout that supports your goals and dreams.

The Big Put-Off

Welcome! We're so glad you're still here. The suburbs, malls, and hospitals are full of people who would NEVER get this far into a conversation about fitness. So, thank you for allowing us to spend some time with you and hopefully, and quite intentionally, encourage you to do something exciting for yourself and those you love.

To do that, we're going to have to break out the dreaded word: "fitness". If your teeth are clenched, your eyebrows are furrowed, or a sense of dread is moving over you like a heavy blanket at the mere thought of walking into a health club, you're not alone. Lots of people are putting off taking care of their health and not entering a gym and we understand why.

As a product of the 60's and 70's, it's likely your idea of fitness comes from visions of Jack LaLanne, Jane Fonda and Tony Horton. Or maybe it's a more recent Saturday morning rock-hard abs celebrity routine where just the warm-up is enough to embarrass you, or worse yet - harm you.

Perhaps you've even tried multiple times to "like fitness", only to experience exercise programs designed for someone half your age who possesses entirely different abilities so that you ended up with a workout that left you feeling old, woefully uncoordinated, and miserable.

No matter how or why, if your idea of "fitness" has been tainted to the point that you've put it off way too long, we're here to get you back on track and offer you multiple excuse-busting reasons why now is the time to get moving.

As you proceed, we encourage you to relax and envision something new and better for yourself based on research and techniques specifically designed for mature adults like you who live a more active lifestyle than any other generation in history.

Inside the safe pages of this book we are not going to present you with a message reiterating how "exercise is good for you". We presume you already believe that to be true and you're here to dig deeper into what fitness and exercise could offer you at this stage in life. We ARE going to do our best to help you overcome your fears and unfamiliarity with exercise, and more specifically introduce "functional fitness", so you're excited and comfortable about inviting us to partner with you as your fitness coach.

You probably used to tell your kids to eat their vegetables because they were good for them (and you probably can remember their faces). Since you are reading this book it's a safe bet that you are the type of person who doesn't get really excited about exercise. You don't live to exercise and can probably list at least 20 things you would rather be doing. But you also know deep down inside that you could do those 20 things better if you had more strength, more endurance, better balance, and more energy.

You may have even had something of a wake-up call in your life recently where you've realized you need to change the trajectory of the path you're on.

For many of our clients, those wake up calls are events like a major health challenge of a friend, or their own medical scare; the birth of a grandchild; the trip opportunity of a lifetime; a new relationship (or a broken one), or the realization that taking care of the physical needs of someone they love is going to require more strength and ability from them.

That's why we're here.

As you age, "fitness" becomes more critical to support the things you are passionate about doing…for the rest of your life.

Viewed from that standpoint, fitness becomes something you should cherish.

But not all fitness programs are equal. Many exercises are simply not well designed and are often rather *dysfunctional* with respect to the aging process. Your body's needs at age 50, 60 and beyond are vastly different than your body's needs when you were in your 20s and 30s. Strength and energy are much more important to you than gorgeous abs and a firm tush. Balance - something you didn't think twice about in your youth, is now critical to your safety.

This book is designed to help you discover and appreciate how this new definition of fitness fits into your goals as you age. **The good news is you have a lot of control over how you age, and the right kinds of exercise can make a huge difference.**

Let's explore that idea together.

Chapter 1

Fitness Starts in Your Mind and Your Dreams

You first have to believe that you can be fit, strong and healthy at any age. You must believe that good health is not just a gift for youth, or something relegated to your past. Strength, vitality and vibrancy are gifts for today and for your future. But here is the challenging part... you have some work to do to maintain and build your strength, your vitality and your vibrancy.

Let's face it if you don't value taking care of your body and your physique who will? The choice really is yours. You can live your life to its full vitality, or you can settle for a future that is less than optimal, marked by physical challenges.

Imagine you're on a trip to Rome, standing at the foot of the famous 138 Spanish Steps. Your entire family is along - your kids and your grandkids and you are in one of the most magnificent places in the world. This is a pinnacle moment in your life.

PAUSE. What's your mind telling you <u>right now</u>?

Possibility #1 – You're energized. The sun is out, the air is fresh and you're set for another adventure. You jokingly challenge your grandchildren to a race to the top. With no intention of actually winning, your greatest joy just comes from being the cool grandparent who's still got it. You value being an inspiration and role model to those around you and you use it to benefit others.

Possibility #2 – You're already tired. Your legs are aching from walking most of the day and the idea of climbing even half way up to enjoy the view is exhausting, maybe impossible. Even if you could, you'd be trading that adventure for something else later. You encourage the family to go on while you wait for them. Your gift to them is stepping aside so you're not a burden to their experience. They'll understand. After all, this is what aging looks like. Or perhaps you believe you're becoming a burden and they might be regretting you coming along on the trip. Maybe next time you'll just stay home.

PAUSE. If Possibility #1 is where your mind went first, congratulations. Overcoming an aging mindset is a big hurdle to free yourself up to pursue your vision.

If Possibility #2 is what your brain believes, your first assignment is to start dreaming a new dream. Maybe it's not Rome on your list, maybe it is Disney World, or the Grand Canyon, or just a regular Tuesday morning round of 18 holes of golf with friends - the point is, the moments you still dream of are only fully possible if your brain knows your body is fit for the activity!

We want you to be fit enough to live out your hopes and dreams for years to come with the people you love. This type of fitness is called "Functional Fitness" – the ability of the body to perform, a/k/a function, properly at whatever task is needed. It's a very different type of fitness training.

Functional Fitness is a Gift to You and Your Family

So let's focus on what Functional Fitness can do for you and your family. We'll start with a list of the gifts and then in Chapter 2, we will discuss how we make these available to you.

Gift #1: Improve your "Doability".

In the fitness world, this is called "functional ability" but we like calling it "doability" because you will be able to do the things you already do even better. Your ability to work around the house, volunteer at a food bank, hike through a national park, hit a tennis ball, ski down a mountain, and even tote luggage will improve. And since you'll do it with greater ease and less discomfort, you'll hit the tennis ball harder, ski better, or simply stay out enjoying your day longer. You will even find yourself doing things you haven't done in years because you couldn't do them anymore or trying new things you never thought you could do "at your age". Our functional fitness program will build the strength, energy, stamina and flexibility you need for all of life's tasks.

Gift #2: Feel Better.

This improvement in function is accompanied by a reduction in the discomfort and pain often associated with many physical activities. Participants typically report that minor irritations such as knee pain from osteoarthritis or low back pain get notably better. Climbing stairs doesn't hurt as much. Working in the garden doesn't come with as high a price as before. Not to mention you just feel better overall as your body becomes more fit.

Gift #3: Power the Mind.

The neuroscientific research from the past 10 years has made it very clear that a person's mind can improve at any age. Exercise and a healthy diet are two major factors that are important to having a healthy brain. Having a fit and capable body also boosts your self-confidence. You may have never thought about lifting weights for your brain, but recent research is confirming long held beliefs: the stronger you keep your body the stronger and sounder you keep your mind.

Gift #4: Build Muscle.

Wait, before you go there, let me assure you, you will not "bulk up" and look unnatural for your age! With functional fitness, you are not going to grow big bulky muscles or look like a bodybuilder. You will gain muscle and lose body fat, creating a leaner, toned body. However, we're going to intentionally spread your muscle gain throughout different parts of the body - including both the primary and secondary muscle groups.

You'll have power and strength everywhere you need it, not just in the 'vanity parts' emphasized by weightlifters and body builders. You'll be fit and toned. More importantly, you will be stronger in a functional way. Muscles can get stronger without getting bigger and our program takes advantage of that process so that you get stronger without much increase in muscle size.

Gift #5: Less Injury.

"Boomeritis" is a term coined by Dr. Nicholas A. DiNubile, an orthopedic surgeon, in 1999 while trying to explain the explosion in joint and muscle problems in people in their 40's and 50's. When aging joints meet traditional exercise programs, the result is often injury and/or pain. Our Functional Aging Training model helps to prevent injury that can occur from exercise, sport, work or daily activities because it helps to improve the accuracy and efficiency of human movement rather than just focusing on building a particular muscle.

To put it frankly, your exercise program should not be injuring you, or making your joints hurt more. Just the opposite in fact. It should make you more injury resistant and help your joints feel better. Our training program will lead to a leaner, stronger, more coordinated, balanced body which means you will reduce your risk of injuries and joint problems down the road.

Gift #6: Better Balance.

Better balance is a great and intentional benefit of our program. By including a wide variety of stances and body positions in addition to movements that specifically challenge gait, balance improves significantly. This means a reduced risk of falling and a greater ability to tackle activities that require good balance. It means you will still be able to navigate those rugged trails you enjoy hiking and take off on an unknown adventure knowing you have the balance and coordination to handle whatever lies ahead.

Gift #7: Quality of Life and Maybe Longevity

Exercise is a powerful stimulus that can keep you fit, healthy, strong, independent, vibrant, engaged and functional well into late-life. Exercise may add years to your life but, more importantly, it will add life to your years. And it is never too late to start. No matter how many years you have in your rear-view mirror, you still have many more down the road in front of you and you want those years to be the best that they can possibly be. After all, you've paid your dues (and your taxes), learned your lessons, worked hard, climbed the ladder, raised children and given of yourself. And you want to keep doing all of those things you still enjoy and even try some things you've always wanted to do but just couldn't find the time to fit it in.

Ready to Handle Life

You now stand at the pinnacle of life, looking over the precipice at a new adventure. Your mind and your spirit are up for the challenge but you wonder if your body can handle it. You don't quite have the pep in your step that you used to. There are a few more aches and pains in your joints. Some of the tasks that used to be easy are now a little more difficult for you or you may be avoiding them altogether.

It's like it says in the *Old Folks Boogie* by the band Little Feat (Barrere, 1977), "When your mind makes a promise that your body can't fill." The aging process is taking its toll. Combine that with years of not exercising and the effects are magnified.

There are things you want to do but wonder if your body will allow you to. Whether it's climbing the Temple of the Sun at Machu Picchu, enjoying a bike tour in Holland, spending a day at the zoo with your grandchildren, dancing the night away to your favorite music, or simply taking care of your garden, your body needs to be ready for the challenge. We believe you should be dancing at your grandchildren's weddings, not just sitting there as a quiet observer.

Now you can begin to see why working with trainers who are specialists in fitness for specific types of functionality is important to you. The industry term is "Functional Fitness".

For the past 30+ years, the fitness industry by and large has been focused on youth, vanity, weight loss and the glamourous side of fitness – ignoring the elements of fitness with respect to successful aging. In contrast, Functional Fitness experts focus on fitness movements or programs that lead to greater enhancement in performance, or human function.

A leading authority on Functional Fitness as people age across the life span is the Functional Aging Institute. FAI is an educational and certifying body for fitness professionals around the world. It's an amazing and exciting movement created to empower the greatest population of people entering the third phase of their life together – so-called "Baby Boomers".

At its very core, our vision as Functional Aging Specialists is to help this population to do what they WANT to do, what they NEED to do, and what they enjoy or even DREAM of doing with greater ease, less pain, and higher levels of proficiency.

Understanding what's possible for the Boomer generation based on new research and technology is energizing!

As certified Functional Aging Specialists, we believe:

- Aging is a normal process...but growing old is optional.

- Improving functional fitness is critical to living a long, healthy and enjoyable life.

- Traditional resistance training does NOT maximize function.

- It is NEVER too late to begin a fitness program and reap its benefits.

- If you move better, you will feel better. If you feel better, you will move more. If you move more, you will look better.

- Fitness is one of the best investments of time, money and effort that a mature adult can make and it will yield huge benefits.

- All exercise programs are NOT created equal!

Our mission is to help people achieve the best possible health and quality of life through innovative and evidence-based functional fitness programs that are safe, effective, enjoyable and purposeful.

Chapter 2

Functional Fitness for Mature Adults

There is a lot of bad information about exercise being passed around today, *especially* when it comes to mature adults. As certified Functional Aging Specialists, we've worked hard to achieve a greater degree of training, experience, and expertise on the process of exercise and aging for the benefit of our clients.

We cringe when we see "expert trainers" on TV shows and even in our community sharing advice that is misinformed at best and absolutely awful at worst. We're fearful when we spot bad (even dangerous) advice dispensed confidently as fitness training. Even a simple weight lifting motion appropriate for a 35 year old could cause a severe shoulder injury in someone a few years older. We urge you to do your homework because the fitness industry is largely unregulated. ONLY trust your health to people who care enough to pursue constant education *and certification* to care for your needs.

Designed to Get Results You Want and Need

One of the primary challenges of the aging process is the natural loss of muscle mass and strength, a process called sarcopenia. Sarcopenia is exacerbated by an inactive lifestyle.

Scientists have been studying sarcopenia for decades. The original thinking was that loss of strength was inevitable with aging. A landmark study by Fiatarone and Singh in the early 1990's showed that heavy resistance training for even 90-100 year olds was safe and effective for improving muscle mass and strength. Yes, 90 to 100 year olds!

The report said that by following traditional progressive resistance training, older adults can increase their muscular strength anywhere from 25% to more than 100% depending on the exercise program being used, the duration of the training, age and gender of the client, and the specific muscle groups being trained. They recommended mature adults engage in at least two days per week of moderate intensity strength training that includes 8-10 exercises involving the major muscle groups.

And that's where the confusion began.

Gyms at that point were designed for vanity body building and loaded with weight-lifting machines. Women-friendly gyms started springing up in competition, including ladies circuit gyms and Curves-type centers; but again the emphasis was on a circuit of machines. The advantages of using gym machines are that they are pretty easy to learn and use independently, they're somewhat "dummy" proof, and they isolate the muscle group being worked. Unfortunately it's this idea of muscle isolation from the world of bodybuilding that has embedded itself into the larger world of fitness. The point is to get into a contraption (typically in a seated position) that places almost all of the work on the targeted muscle and allows the rest of the body to relax. Since that one muscle is doing all of the work, it is going to increase its size and strength quicker. And guess what? It works. If your goal is to improve the size and strength of one particular muscle group then this is a great way to do it.

It is this type of muscle isolation program that has been used in many exercise studies with mature adults including the one cited above. In fact the research has been overwhelming: men and women at any age and in just about any health condition can get stronger and grow their muscles even after age 90.

Unfortunately, researchers hypothesized that as people got stronger, functional outcomes would follow. But they did not! Thankfully, researchers started shifting towards evaluating the *functional effects* of resistance exercise (weight lifting) and the evidence is quite surprising. Startling in fact!

"You missed it by that much!"
– Maxwell Smart

This is where the value of the Functional Aging Institute training gets most interesting for you.

Until recently the fitness industry has really missed the mark on fitness programming for the mature adult. The Functional Aging Institute highlights some key studies published in 2001, 2004, and 2008 which critically evaluate the relationship between the improvement of factors such as strength, joint range of motion, aerobic capacity, body composition, etc. following training with measures of function such as gait speed, chair rise time, stair climbing, balance and weighted lifting tasks. They all concluded the same thing – the relationship is not nearly as strong as we always assumed it to be.

In 2001, one group of authors specifically noted that subjects who improved the most on strength were not necessarily the ones who improved the most on the functional measures.[1] Another group of authors (2004) concluded that strength gains do not equate to similar functional gains[2]. More recently, an extensive review of the research (Orr et al. 2008) determined that there is limited evidence to show that the best strength training protocols still are unable to improve balance performance in older adults.[3]

Don't miss the impact of what this tells us. It is hard for body builder fans to swallow, but the evidence is pretty clear:

Stronger is not always better!

Traditional muscle-isolation type resistance exercise programs will significantly improve strength but will probably NOT significantly improve physical function. What this means is that traditional forms of strength training may NOT actually help you move better, and do the things you want to do easier. This has led some researchers to declare that novel approaches are needed!

---

[1] Keysor JJ, Jette AM. *Have we oversold the benefit of late-life exercise?* J Gerontol A Biol Sci Med Sci. 2001 Jul;56(7):M412-23.

[2] Latham, Bennet, Stretton, Anderson. Systematic Review of Progressive Resistance Strength Training in Older Adults. J Gerontol A Biol Sci Med Sci(2004) 59 (1): M48-M61

[3] Orr R, Raymond J, Singh M F. Efficacy of progressive resistance training on balance performance in older adults: a systematic review of randomized controlled trials. Sports Medicine 2008; 38(4): 317-343

At the other end of the spectrum, there have been plenty of 'novel approaches' that also haven't translated into functional ability as hoped. Swinging to the oldies with Richard Simmons, group Jazzercise, or joining your friends for a 30-minute training circle may make for fun workouts for a while, but they only touch on the surface level of endurance and muscle strength. To relate it to the medical world, it's the difference between taking your health concerns to the nearest general practitioner or seeing a doctor who specializes in your ailment with a proven track record of success.

The philosophies, principles, strategies and techniques that are used in the Functional Aging Training Model are the keys to improving physical function. **Most of the fitness industry and the average personal trainer are still using antiquated concepts of training for mature clients!** All exercise programs are not equal, and you can't just compare them on cost, location, or locker room amenities. If you really want results that are going to change your life and change your outlook on your future you cannot afford to make the mistake of thinking all gyms are equal and all trainers are basically the same.

It is critical that you read, understand and put functional principles into action. In the next chapter, we will outline how our philosophy is different, and how it is grounded in research and scientific evidence, and honed with real world experience.

If you want to start moving better, feeling better and looking better, then you have to train appropriately for your age and ability. Whether you are new to fitness or have been exercising your whole life, we'll help you discover an approach to exercise that is vastly different than what you will see in 95%

of the gyms out there. You will finally understand how to train your body to get results that are both relevant for you now and that will help prepare you to remain functional as you get older.

As a champion for your own health, you're going to look and feel much better inside and out.

You're going to have the strength and energy to do the things you love to do better and more often.

And equally important, you're going to give the people around you - including your spouse, your family, your friends, or your community - the gift of enjoying life with you.

Let's get started!

Chapter 3

Discovering a New Kind of Fitness

At Westminster Fit Body our fitness program is much more than just an exercise program. It's a formula specifically crafted by the Functional Aging Institute through years of research and testing. This is why we place a high value on being a Functional Aging Specialist and why we've chosen to model a training philosophy that has been developed by the leaders in the industry for aging and exercise. The benefit for you is a proven system of training that is incredibly effective, efficient and safe.

Working with us, you'll discover we value:

- An in-depth UNDERSTANDING of the aging process and its implications for your exercise program.

- A RECOGNITION of the desires, goals and aspirations that are specific to you and your dreams.

- A strong BELIEF that people can be fit, healthy, vibrant and functional at any age.

- An APPROACH to exercise that is grounded in evidence and honed with experience.

Our Key Foundations

In the field of exercise science there are some known principles that have been shown to produce results in performance. We follow two key principles that form the foundation of everything we will do with you.

This means we won't just pick an exercise because we saw it in a magazine, or thought it looked cool. Every exercise we offer is grounded in our two foundational principles: the concepts of specificity and the concept of progressive overload. These concepts are supposed to be foundational to all exercise programs, but are often forgotten or overlooked when it comes to mature clients.

The **CONCEPT OF SPECIFICITY states that how a person trains determines the type of gains they make.** Simply stated, "How you train is how you gain." This means that the kinds of exercises a person performs, and how they perform them will determine the type and magnitude of results that the person sees. This principle is obvious when we consider someone who starts a walking program because they want to improve the strength of their arms. Even to the untrained eye this doesn't make sense. Walking may be a good choice for improving cardiovascular endurance and decreasing health risks but it has virtually no impact at all on arm strength. It is the wrong type of program for the desired results.

If you are like most mature adults, you would say that one of the most important results that you would like to see from exercise is increased physical function. Put more simply, you want to be able to move better and easier with less discomfort and pain. Whether that means playing golf or tennis, traveling, enjoying hobbies, playing with grandchildren, performing yard work, or whatever it is you enjoy doing, you want to be able to do those things with greater ease and less pain.

Our program is focused very specifically on increasing physical function. Therefore, every technique, every method, and every exercise is designed to get you to your goals. When you're achieving your goals, you're excited, satisfied and rewarded. We want that for all of our clients, so you'll see that we spend time with you to discover your goals and what you need from your fitness program to accomplish them. We enjoy helping you achieve even the most specific of goals!

The CONCEPT OF PROGRESSIVE OVERLOAD states that the body must continually be challenged with more difficult tasks or exercises in order for it to continue to adapt and grow. The body will adapt only to the level of challenge that you give it and will not improve any more until it is given a greater challenge. There are lots of ways to progressively overload the body such as lifting heavier weights, completing more repetitions, performing the exercise for a longer period of time (e.g. jogging for 30 minutes instead of 20), increasing the intensity, or making a movement more complex. We'll use a myriad of methods, many of which you will rarely see used by most trainers, to continually overload the body's systems so that you continue to make improvements.

By those standards, it's troublesome to see so many traditional trainers repeating the same circuits or operate with a belief that hitting a plateau is "good enough" for an older person. Uneducated and mis-informed, they're scared they're going to *hurt* you so they stop *helping* you.

We believe you're stronger than that and we want you to make constant progress – getting better and better as you age! So yes, you can be absolutely sure we will be progressively increasing the challenge, and encouraging you to surprise even yourself.

Mixing Things Up Ensures Better Results

So just how are we going to ensure your results? We are going to train all the components of your body you need to function!

Our goal is to help you **Move Better**, which will help you **Move More**, which will help you **Feel Better**.

It really is that simple, however how we will accomplish that is a bit more complex. Everything has a purpose and we're going to manipulate variables such as body position, stance, arm position, arm movement patterns, direction, distance, depth, velocity, equipment and complexity in a purposeful manner in order to create exercise movements that will accomplish our goal of improving physical function (the concept of specificity). These exercise movements are then further "tweaked" (by mixing up the variables) in a highly-ordered process to ensure that you are progressively challenged as you improve your functional fitness (progressive overload). This means as you start to move better, we will make it more complex so you improve even more.

If you want to go take an adventurous hike, you really don't know how many complex movements might be required. We want to be sure you are ready for all of them so you can really thrive in that hiking environment. If you imagine all the various tweaks and changes you might have to make on a rigorous outdoor hike...over a tree, under a tree, across a stream, up onto a boulder, change in terrains, uphill, downhill, you have to make numerous tweaks in your movement patterns. That's why we will always be making meaningful purposeful tweaks in our time together too.

These "tweaks" allow us to create a continuum of functional challenge. We can change just one variable to either bump up the challenge just a little bit or to refocus the exercise movement to work on a different component of function altogether. We can also change multiple variables simultaneously to significantly increase the functional demand. The combinations are almost limitless. This complexity of progressions is why working with a fitness professional will ensure that your results will be significant. This is great news for you because the programs will never get boring or routine!

For example, consider how some simple variations in a standing rowing movement can alter the demands placed on the core and trunk. We may start with a standing, split-stance (one foot slightly ahead of the other), two-arm row using resistance tubing. In this position the trunk is being pulled forward creating a large front-to-back plane demand. This causes the muscles on the back of the body to really work to keep the body in an upright position. However, by dropping out the left hand and only using the right hand to perform the rowing movement we can change the demand on the trunk. Instead of a front-to-back plane demand there is now a rotational plane demand because only one hand is holding the resistance which creates an imbalance between the right and left sides. Instead of being pulled forward, the trunk is pulled into rotation (twisting) which it must resist. This completely changes the muscle activation in the back and hips. We can further increase the challenge by adding a backwards lunge to this movement. So now the person must step backwards with the right leg into a lunge position while simultaneously performing a tubing row with the right hand. Not only does this require a lot more lower-body strength it is also a more complicated movement which requires much more motor control, coordination and balance to perform.

This is just one simple example of how small and seemingly insignificant changes in the variables of an exercise movement can create important differences in the demands on the body. These manipulations are embedded throughout our sessions and although we want you to understand the philosophy and approach behind the workouts, the great thing is that you don't have to think about it. We've done all of the work for you by creating workouts that are extremely well-balanced and focused.

A Purpose for Every Exercise

As we age, muscle coordination decreases, balance worsens, agility declines, strength and power decrease. The list goes on. You must be training all components of your movements to protect and develop your muscle strength, mobility, coordination, posture, agility, balance, etc. You can't do that by simply walking on a treadmill or doing some weight training.

We also know you have a limited amount of time and energy to devote to an exercise program, so every exercise should have a specific purpose. You can ask us at any moment during a session, "Why are you doing this particular exercise for me at this point in my training program?" There should be a solid purpose for every exercise movement and every variation that is used and, if not, we should reevaluate it. You don't want to waste your time performing exercises that have minimal value toward helping you accomplish your goals.

For example if sit-ups serve you no purpose (and for most of our clients that is the case) why would we ever have you do them? The long-held myth of the well-rounded routine is entrenched in our minds. The myth states that a good routine is one that is well-balanced and includes exercises for "every major muscle group." But the best routines are not balanced, they are prioritized. Older men with a background in carpentry, gardening, or a related area typically have very strong forearms and arms. Those that are or were significantly overweight often have very strong calf muscles. And the list goes on. Think about it. Wouldn't it make more sense to target the weakest areas first before spending time and energy on an area that is doing just fine?

Break away from the constraints of the "well-rounded routine" and stop wasting your time and energy performing exercises that do not serve your individual needs and goals. With us, you always have the flexibility to swap out exercises that you feel might be more appropriate for you. After all, we're here to serve you for your goals.

Real Life Moves in all 3 Planes

Life is three-dimensional. You reach, bend, lean, turn, twist, stoop and change directions constantly throughout your day. In essence, you continually face challenges from the front-to-back, side-to-side and rotational planes – these are the three planes of human movement.

Side-to-Side Plane: Side-to-side movement or force. Shuffling sideways, arm raises to the side, side-bending or leg raises to the side (even when you are lying down) are all side-to-side plane movements. Holding a heavy bag in one hand by your side, while standing, is an example of a side-to-side plane force.

Front-to-Back or Back-to-Front Plane: Frontward or backward movement or force. Walking forward or backward, sit-ups, standing up, arm raises to the front and rowing are all front-to-back plane movements. If you were in a standing position and someone was pushing on your chest that would be an example of a front to back plane force because, even though you aren't moving, your muscles have to resist to keep you from falling backwards. If someone were pushing on your back then that would be a back to front plane force.

Rotational Plane: Twisting movement or force. This could be rotating or twisting your upper body while your lower body stays in place, twisting your lower body while your upper body stays in place or moving both (either in the same or opposite directions) simultaneously. It can also include a force that wants you to rotate but that you resist against.

Train movements before muscles

As we discussed earlier, traditional strength training exercises offer some benefits for combating sarcopenia (loss of muscle mass due to age), building strength, and, to a lesser degree, improving function. So it is erroneous to conclude that these exercises are not functional at all. Even arm curls are functional to a certain degree because you have to use your biceps to lift or pull objects. It is better to view exercises along a functional continuum with some exercises being more functional and some being less functional.

We will always be striving to move towards more complex functional movement patterns as you progress. This means we will work on putting more simple movements together over time. For example if we want to work on a floor to overhead press movement (lifting a weight from the floor to over head) we might first master the overhead press from a standing position. Then we might master bending over and picking up a weight, and then put them all together into the more complex movement.

Stand Up, Stay Up

Mobility is a critical component for your continued health and longevity. Loss of mobility can lead to a downward "death spiral" of declining health and activity levels. But beyond the decreased mobility is a critical component of life satisfaction. **Loss of mobility usually means loss of independence.** People can no longer work, shop, play, or do household chores because they cannot get up and around to do them. They then end up relying on help from others. **Related to this is the risk of falling.** Falls are a significant threat to the mature population, often leading to hospitalization, the need for long-term care and are even the leading cause of accidental death.

So because we know that as you age your ability and agility on your feet is so vital to long term health we will do the majority of our exercise program standing. Mobility and balance are best improved in standing positions. The standing position utilizes many more muscle groups than sitting and is a more complex neuromuscular challenge that requires greater degrees of strength, proprioception, center of gravity control and postural stability.

Seated exercise may be purposeful when:

- You become fatigued.
- You are not yet ready for higher-level progressions or you are too unstable on your feet.
- The movement involves sit-to-stand transitions.

Complicated First, Simple Last

During the course of an exercise training session it is typical for clients to tire out as both muscle and mental fatigue set in. For mature clients this loss of energy and focus can create potentially dangerous scenarios and increase risk of injury. The longer the session continues, the greater the likelihood that attention and performance will wane. Since we are aware of this natural decline in energy, we will have you perform more complicated tasks earlier in the session while you are still physcially and mentally fresh.

More complicated movements include dynamic balance tasks, gait variations, agility drills (ladder, dot, obstacles) and multi-planar movements. The latter parts of the session would be more appropriate for isolated strength training, seated movements and floor work.

Safety First….But No Kid Gloves

Getting off the traditional exercise machines in order to perform dynamic, multi-dimensional exercises of increasing complexity can bring with it an increase in the risk of falling and injury. Therefore, we will always take the appropriate measures to ensure safety while maximizing the potential for success.

First off, we will need you to be honest about your current level of health and physical ability. Although we want you to step out of your comfort zone and put as much as you can into your workouts, we also want you to be safe.

If you have significant health concerns such as cardiovascular disease, joint replacements, diabetes, osteoporosis or similar conditions then we will modify your program accordingly.

The primary safety concern we see is the risk of a client falling. Many of the movements we use will either rely on good balance (and stability) or will purposefully challenge balance. We will often position you so that you have a chair, table, or railing to rely on if you need it and we'll make sure your environment is free of trip hazards. Our goal is to dramatically improve balance and coordination, but to do that in a safe way, not in a manner that puts you in danger or at risk.

Most importantly, we will be right here with you every step of the way, monitoring your progress as you complete each fitness task.

Chapter 4

Functional Fitness Equipment

Seeing a gym filled with equipment can feel intimidating, so let's spend a few minutes going through what you can expect when you work out with us.

When you walk out into our fitness area, you'll see lots of functional fitness equipment. Our space is split into two sections- the BLACK plyo mat contains our suspension trainers (TRX and APT), a tool we use that supports the use of your core at all times yet accommodates for individual imbalances and fitness levels. We love the TRX for it's unique adjustability to support joint issues; however we do not recommend them for everyone! As you move toward the RED carpet springloaded floor you'll see our free weights and other functional fitness gear. This unique floor is great on joints as it counterbalances your weight, provides a little bit of instability to support core strength through all movements and is comfortable to kneel and lay down on.

For functional fitness training, equipment is kept to a

minimum but may include resistance tubing, dumbbells, a step (or stair), or an exercise mat. Many exercises only utilize body weight. **By keeping equipment to a minimum we maximize your use of your body weight and develop your total body functional strength.** Again, it really isn't about the equipment as much as about the techniques and the progressions. We believe the most important piece of equipment is the one you carry with you everywhere you go. Since some of the equipment and movement patterns will be new to you, we will highlight just a few of them here so you will be prepared and comfortable. If this equipment is unfamiliar to you then read the descriptions below.

Resistance Tubing/Anchor Point/Rip Trainer

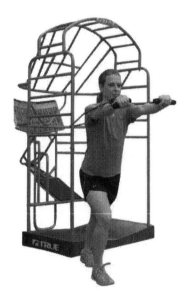

These functional tools allow us to generate resistance from an anchor point, and not rely on gravity. This allows us to have resistance at varying angles and positions for pulling, pushing and rotational movements. These pieces of equipment are essential for certain movements where we can't use dumbbells or other weighted implements. They are also great for traveling or when you can't make it in for a training session. We can help you find a quality one for home or travel use. Here are a couple of simple tips for when we ask you to use this form of resistance.

Tip #1: Move to Adjust Resistance – When performing an exercise movement with tubing and/or bungies, you may find that it is either too easy or too difficult. A quick way to adjust the resistance is to either move closer to the anchor (making the movement easier) or to move further away from the anchor (making the movement more difficult). Make these adjustments quickly and remember that the last few repetitions of each exercise need to be challenging for you or you will not be getting the most benefit out of it.

Tip #2: Control in Both Directions – Since tubing and/or bungies are elastic they tend to "snap back" when you pull them. It is important that you control the movement in both directions. Do not allow it to "snap back" but rather use slow and controlled movements. When you are done with the exercise, don't just let the tubing go if it is still stretched because it will fly around and hit something or possibly someone standing nearby.

Dumbbells

There are several common mistakes that we'll help you avoid when using dumbbells in your workouts. Avoiding these errors will ensure that you are being safe with the dumbbells and using them properly in order to get the most benefit out of your program.

Mistake #1: Ignoring the Laws of Gravity - Dumbbells 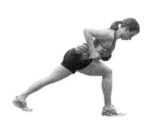 are gravity-based equipment. Since gravity pulls objects down to the ground then that means dumbbells need to move in line with the pull of gravity in order to work properly. So any exercise using dumbbells needs to move them primarily up and down (perpendicular to the floor). Any exercise movement that moves the dumbbells parallel to the floor is not using them properly. This is why dumbbells and resistance bands cannot always be swapped out for a particular exercise with the same result. For example, if you are performing a standing row with tubing, you cannot substitute dumbbells without also changing your body position. In order to use dumbbells in a rowing movement, you would need to lean over so that your trunk is facing the ground. In this position you can use the force of gravity and make Isaac Newton proud.

Mistake #2: Too Much Swing – When any exercise becomes difficult or when your muscles become tired there is a tendency to "cheat." One of the common cheating movements when using dumbbells is swinging the weights instead of lifting them in a slow and controlled fashion. By swinging the weights into the movement, momentum is created which helps you perform the movement but doesn't accomplish the primary goal of working the muscle and increases the risk of accident or injury. Whenever possible, use slow and controlled movements with dumbbells. If you cannot complete the number of repetitions with good form, then simply drop to a lighter dumbbell in order to finish the set. However, there are some exercise movements using resistance tubing that we will have you do as quickly as possible in order to work on muscle power. Make sure you still use good form when performing these kinds of exercises.

Mistake #3: Easy Cheesy – It is imperative that you use dumbbells that are challenging for you when completing the number of repetitions for a particular movement. We have seen, far too often in our experience, that people tend to stick with the same weight for a variety of movements even when they could use a heavier one. Different muscle groups are stronger than others and thus require heavier dumbbells. Don't be afraid to use a heavier weight for a particular exercise. One good way to judge this is to honestly ask yourself if you could have completed a couple more repetitions with good form beyond what the set called for. So if you performed a set of 12 repetitions but could have done 2 more with good form, then it is time to bump up the weight a little. When performing multiple sets, be sure to use the appropriate weight. Don't just go light so you can complete 2 or 3 sets easily. It is okay to have sets 1 and 2 be heavier and set 3 a little lighter due to fatigue.

Medicine Balls

A medicine ball is a weighted ball that's perfect for performing many functional exercises. Just like resistance tubing and dumbbells, there are a few things we'll cover to make using them safe and effective.

Tip #1 - Make sure you are aware if you are using a medicine ball that bounces or one that does not. Not all medicine balls are made equal either, some bounce much more than others, so before you go slamming a ball into the floor only to have it rebound and break your nose, be sure you know what you are working with.

Tip #2 - Make sure you use the appropriate weight. Medicine balls can range from 2 lbs-40 lbs. Be sure you are using one that challenges you, but you can still safely control so you don't hurt yourself or others.

Tip #3 - Remember it is a ball, which means it may bounce, it may roll, it may have a mind of its own at times!

While it is a weighted implement like a dumbbell, it could roll and bounce away or into others, so be careful and mindful of the your safety and the safety of others.

Chapter 5

What to Expect in Your Training Sessions

This chapter will outline what you might experience in a training session. We find that our new clients, particularly those who are completely new to working with a trainer, like to know what they can expect before they step through our door. Thus, these pictures and guides are an example of some of the things you can expect, but not a be-all, end-all list. If you like surprises, you can skip this chapter.

We will design an optimal workout schedule based on your needs and goals. If you need to lose 50 lbs or more, it might be best for you to train with us THREE times per week and also focus on a healthy meal plan. You will be with the trainer for 30 minutes but we ask that you come in 10 – 15 minutes before your session as we will also put together an individual pre-workout routine that should take only 5 – 10 minutes to prepare your body and support some of your individual areas of need.

It's important to explain that there are no perfect or "normal" exercise routines when it comes to functional fitness. Your training sessions are always changing, always progressing and always staying specific for your needs. Remember the principle of progressive overload, so we actually say that the workout that may be perfect for you this week could be rather useless to you in about 2 weeks!

Functional Fitness Movements

On the following pages, we have included a variety of exercise movements we use so you can see what to expect and use this to help reinforce some of the movement patterns on your own.

Woodchops

Rotations with Reach

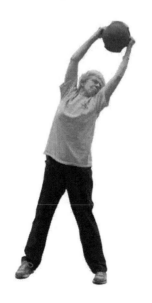
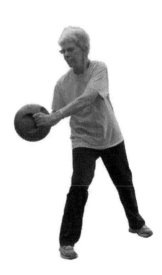

Single Arm Row in a Lunge

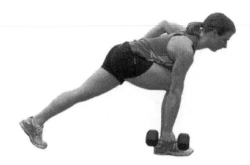

Crossover Reach in Lunge Stance

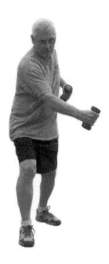

Arm Curls in Lunge Stance

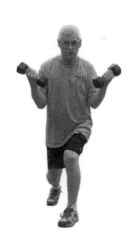

Front Plank with Alternating Leg Raise

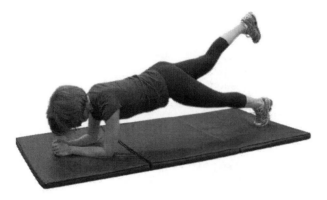

Front Plank with Alternating Arm Raise

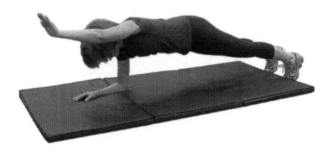

Mountain Climbers

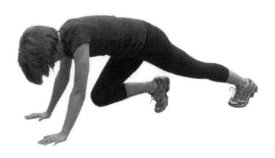

Curl to Press in Lunge Stance

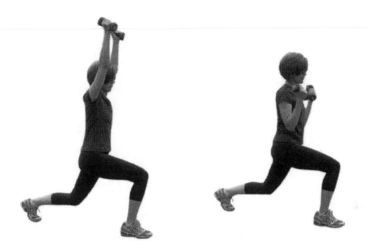

Sit to Stand with Arms Overhead

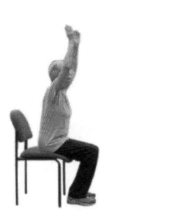
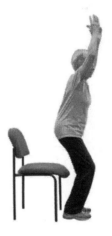

Side Plank with Leg Lift

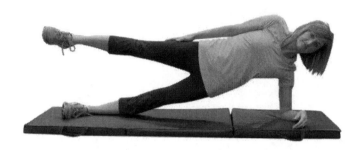

Side Lunge with Overhead Dumbbell Press

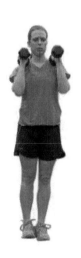 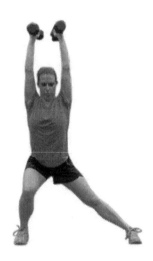

Plank Up-Downs

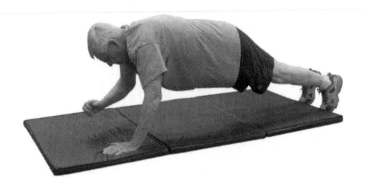

Get Ups with Dumbbell

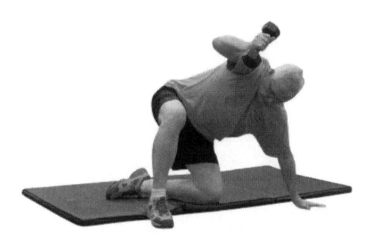

Leg Curl with Ball

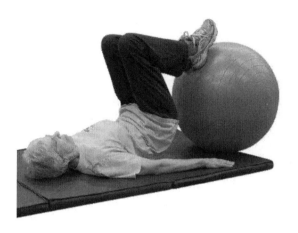

Straight Leg Lift with Ball

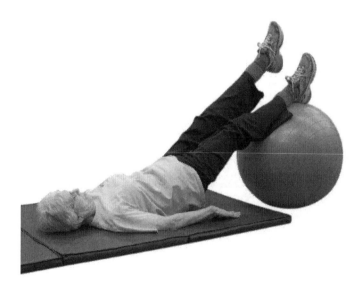

Single-Leg Stiff-Legged Deadlift

Standing Lunge with Dumbbell Overhead Press

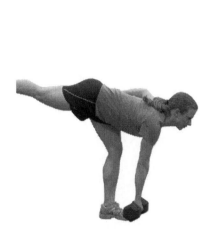

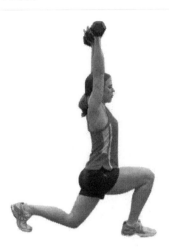

Reverse Crossover Punch with Dumbbell

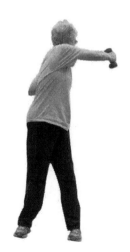

Common Routines

In the previous chapter we explained that we will start you with a beginner routine and then build from there. If a movement is clearly too easy, we will progress to a more appropriate challenge. We will increase the challenge in a variety of ways: we may ask you to perform more repetitions per exercise, add a second set of the exercise, increase the weight or we may move on to a more complex exercise. Another way to make the workouts more challenging is to shorten your rest in between each exercise, so you are moving from exercise to exercise as quickly as possible without rest breaks. Since safety is one of the key principles of training, it is extremely important to us that you perform all exercises in a safe and correct manner. That's why we are right here with you as you learn and perform each task. Along the same lines, we will teach you how to be sure you are ready to begin a training session by being properly warmed up and ready to go.

The majority of our training sessions will be 30 minutes in length. You will see that some of the sample routines for beginners are even shorter than that starting out. The following are a couple of sample beginner training sessions and a couple of intermediate sessions to give you an idea of what to expect. Of course, in reality your sessions will be always changing based on your needs, so these are just some general samples. We don't expect that you will know all the exercises named, and we certainly don't expect that you know how to do them. We will teach you all of these over time.

Functional Warm-up for Beginners

Time: 4-5 min
20-30 seconds of each movement

Woodchops straight up and down
Woodchops down-left to up-right
Woodchops down-right to up-left
March in place
Heel Kicks
Small Forward Lunge with 2-arm reach alternating legs
Small Forward Lunge with 1-arm crossover reach alternating legs and arms
Backwards Lunge with 2-arm overhead reach
March in place
Heel Kicks

Beginner Workout #1

Time: 16-20 min

Chair Stands – 15 reps
Tandem Walk – 30 seconds
Two arm standing shoulder press – 15 reps
Standing two arm tubing row – 15 reps
Heel Walk – 30 seconds

Standing two arm tubing chest press - 15 reps
Kneeling two arm lat pull down – 15 reps
Crossover Walk – 30 seconds
Step Ups right leg – 15 reps
Step Ups left leg – 15 reps

Calf raise (on step or floor) – 15 reps
Bridge – 3 reps (5 sec hold)
Bird Dog – 2 reps each limb (5 sec hold)

Beginner Workout #2

Time: 17-22 min

Split Squat – 12 reps each leg
Sleeping Dog front and back – 3 reps each leg
Two arm standing dumbbell lateral raises – 12 reps
(repeat)

Standing alternating tubing rows – 12 reps each arm
Sleeping Dog side to side – 5 reps
Standing alternating chest press – 12 reps each arm
(repeat)

Standing alternating lat pull down – 12 reps each arm
Heel Toe Rocks – 30 seconds
Side Step Ups – 12 reps each leg
(repeat)

Bridge with arms together – 3 reps (5 sec hold)
Bird Dog with limb movement to side – 2 reps each limb
(repeat)

Functional Warm-up for Intermediate & Advanced

Time: 4-5min
30-40 seconds of each exercise

Marches with torso twist (elbow to knee)
Heel Kicks with side step and squat
Split Squat right leg
Split Squat left leg
Hand Walks
Mountain Climbers
Backward Lunges with twist alternating legs

Intermediate Workout #1

Time: 16 min

Stationary Lunge – 12 reps each leg
Bush Walk – 30 seconds
Standing upright tubing row – 12 reps

Standing reciprocating row – 12 reps each arm
Monster Walk – 30 seconds
Standing reciprocating chest press – 12 reps each arm

Stationary Lunge – 12 reps each leg
Bush Walk – 30 seconds
Standing upright tubing row – 12 reps

Standing reciprocating row – 12 reps each arm
Monster Walk – 30 seconds
Standing reciprocating chest press – 12 reps each arm

Half-kneeling reciprocating lat pull down -12 reps each arm
High kicks – 30 seconds
Step Ups with knee lift – 12 reps each leg

Front Plank on knees – 10 seconds
Side Plank on knees – 10 seconds each side

Front Plank on knees – 10 seconds
Side Plank on knees – 10 seconds

Iso twists with tubing – 2 reps each side (10 sec hold)

Intermediate Workout #2
Time: 16-20 min

Stationary Lunge with reach – 12 reps each leg
Carioche Step – 20 seconds
Standing 1 arm tubing shoulder press – 12 reps each arm
(repeat)

Standing 1 arm row – 12 reps each arm
Under the Rope – 20 seconds
Standing 1 arm chest press – 12 reps each arm
(repeat)

Standing reciprocating lat pull down – 12 reps each arm
Straight leg march – 20 seconds
Step ups with knee and arm raise – 12 reps each leg

Reverse planks – 10 seconds
Side plank from knees – 10 seconds each side
(repeat)

Standing iso tubing hold with press outs – 10 seconds each side
(repeat)

Now that we have given you a taste and sample of what some of your exercise sessions might look like, let's recap and review. First keep in mind that your safety is our utmost concern. This program is of no use to you if you wind up hurting yourself. Some exercises may not be appropriate for you if you have specific joint or health concerns such as shoulder issues or knee pain. Please do not take the "I'll tough it out approach".

In order to get the most out of any program you need to make purposeful decisions for every aspect of training. Let's talk briefly about what that might mean for you. If you want to be able to get down on the floor to spend more time with your grandchildren and get back up again easily, then exercises related to getting on the floor, being on the floor and getting up from the floor will have more importance for you. However, if you want to hit a golf ball further and with less back pain, then more standing exercises with rotational (twisting) movements will be important. If you are having trouble with balance or have fallen recently, then spending focused time on balance specific exercises may be of most importance for you. The list can be very broad or narrow and specific so the fitness program will be tailored not only to your current ability, but also your dreams, goals and aspirations.

This doesn't mean you will do only the exercises specific to your main goals, but it does mean you will have a program that will focus on those types of exercises or begin to add more of those exercises into your routines. Of course, all of our clients will have their exercise programs changing each week and progressing over time. You do not want to do the same exercise routine over and over and over. We will often be encouraging you to try new movements and new levels of challenge.

After a few weeks to a couple of months, you will notice how far you have come and how much more complex your training program has become. Also keep in mind there are several ways in which we can make even the same exercise routine progressively harder. And we are always accessible if you want additional guidance at home or with any other health-related concern.

For maximal results you need to do the routines consistently with a little bit of variety in the exercise routines from day to day and constantly progressing. It is as simple as saying that if you don't have a plan to progressively challenge yourself then you aren't likely to make much progress. Your consistent attendance week after week for training is vital so we can take you to the next level.

Chapter 6

Preparing

What should you wear?

You don't need to run out and buy an expensive new fitness wardrobe to start training with us, especially when your goal is to reshape and lose weight. Save your shopping dollars for your new body shape!

Clothing: Wear athletic or comfortable clothing that allows complete freedom of movement and allows you to stay cool. Most of our clients wear a comfortable T-shirt or tank top and loose shorts. Women will want a good support or athletic bra. Inspecting your outfit to avoid "wardrobe malfunctions" may also help you feel more comfortable in the variety of positions you may encounter.

Footwear: If you're anxious to make an investment in your wardrobe, great fitting shoes are a good place to start. Most athletic footwear stores will help you make a selection based on your foot shape, gait, and use. New shoes or not, always select athletic shoes with a non-slip sole. (No flats, heels, sandals, flip-flops or slides.) Don't forget socks to protect your skin.

Safety

You need to be aware and always alerting us to any possible health concerns or signs and symptoms. We are trained, but want you to know the list as well.

Signs and Symptoms: If you experience any of the following signs or symptoms during your workout then stop and seek medical attention:

- Dizziness
- Nausea
- Unusual shortness of breath
- Chest pain or tightness
- Pain in neck or jaw or radiating down the left arm
- Lightheadedness

Energy and Well-Being

Perform workouts only when you are well-fueled, hydrated, and well-rested.

Liquids: Have a water bottle handy to sip on during and after your workout to replace the liquids you'll lose due to perspiration. Keeping yourself well hydrated also helps reduce muscle aches. In addition to water, some of our clients like to drink sports drinks. Avoid sugary drinks like sweet tea or soda pop, which will only add empty calories to your diet.

Pre-Workout fuel: Whatever time of day you choose to work out, it's wise to know your body. We suggest most people eat a pre-workout snack or meal 1-2 hours beforehand. Some people do fine on an empty stomach, so be sure to know what works best for you. We do not want you to have a blood sugar crash because you skipped breakfast or lunch.

Post-Workout refueling: After your workout, your body will need to replenish and restore itself so be sure to eat a healthy snack (ideally with some protein) within one hour of finishing your workout.

If you'd like more suggestions on foods and supplements to enhance your workouts, increase your energy levels, and expedite your recovery, be sure to ask us. There are many good options on the market, and of course there are some we recommend above others.

Getting Started

Our programs are designed for you at your current level. There is no minimum "starting" level. We typically tell clients that the first session or two may feel too easy for you as we learn what is most appropriate for your body. Even then, you may still be sore from doing movements your body is not accustomed to performing. Our goal is not to make you sore every time, but with a progressive training program there will be times you will experience some minor muscle soreness. We always, <u>always</u> want to know about joint pain or discomfort that is not muscular. Sometimes we will alter programs or eliminate specific exercises that may be causing you joint pain. There is little to no place for a "no pain, no gain" attitude. We want a solid effort and for you to challenge yourself, but not pain and suffering!

Trust us when we say that in your first week it is SIGNIFICANTLY better to try a workout that is too easy and then move up than it is to attempt a workout that is above your capabilities and possibly get injured or aggravate an existing condition. Remember, discretion is the better part of valor. Many new clients who considered themselves to be fit (and have even worked out regularly in a gym) thought they could easily jump right into an intermediate or advanced level functional workout, but were quickly humbled when it wasn't as easy as they thought. **We will typically err on the side of caution as we ease you in before moving you up to intermediate levels.**

Customized Workouts

Our workout sessions allow for a large degree of customization based on your goals, your dreams, and your aspirations. Exercise movements can be adjusted or substituted to meet your particular needs, conditions, and abilities. While there are many essential components to our programs that can benefit everyone, you may need more strength, or more balance, or more stamina for your goals so we'll customize those areas for you. We also don't want you to shy away from trying new things or getting better at movements that you aren't quite so comfortable with at first, and we will challenge you to do things you may not have even thought possible for your body! We always want you to be listening to what your body is telling you (and of course the advice of your medical professionals,) so don't be afraid to communicate your concern or special requests.

Chapter 7

Inspiring Examples

Fit Body Forever is excited to continue to support clients in their 50's, 60's, 70's, 80's and 90's with their new small group training program. The success stories of the past 7 years are quite impressive!

Building Confidence after an Injury

Here is one of my favorite client stories, since it demonstrates how our best years lie *ahead of* us:

Athletic looking, piercing blue eyes, silver hair, born in 1951: Pam was in her late 50s and had slowed her active lifestyle because of a knee injury and subsequent surgery. After surgery, she continued bicycling and took up daily walking, however, NOT at the pace or endurance she was used to. She had totally given up her favorite endeavors- road running, skiing and

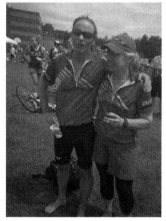 hiking in the beautiful New Hampshire mountains near her home. It seemed as though everything had ground to a halt. Being active was like brushing her teeth- a daily, necessary and consistent part of her life since age twenty-nine. She was afraid of hurting herself again, though, and I didn't blame her.

She reluctantly showed up to one of my 6-week Baby Bootcamp programs, just to try it out. This was a very challenging time for her. I knew I had my work cut out for me as I worked to support Pam in building her "body confidence" up again. We started by strengthening her core, function, flexibility, and endurance.

It worked! Suddenly, Pam was *running* on my spring-loaded floor, squatting, lunging and playing with power moves! Six years later, she is still a part of my regular bootcamp training community. No more "baby bootcamp" for this amazing woman! She participates in the Prouty 100-mile bike race every year!

This past summer, Pam's husband, Jim, decided to try us out to deal with his own injuries sustained from years of being an active athlete. He too, has benefitted from bootcamp training and now, besides their continued participation in the aforementioned century ride, this couple pursues new goals together.

Isn't that great? They are my heroes! - **Pam (65)**

Build It and They Will Come

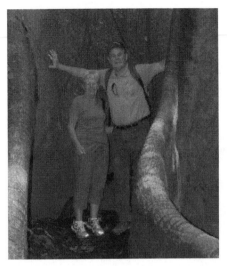

Do you have someone in your life who believes in you more than do you do in yourself? Well that is Pat Boylan to me. When opening up my own space to physically train large groups was just a dream, Pat (my landlord) helped me make it a reality. I remember his words as he showed me the available 4000 sq foot space for my wellness program so clearly. He said "Build it, they will come." And he was right. I never looked back and I will forever be grateful for his confidence in me. There came a time when it was my turn to support him in making his health a priority using the Fit Body Formula.

Pat has been and still is a successful businessman (although we are working on what retirement will look like.) When we initially talked about his goals he mentioned focusing on overall health and stamina and was only 5 on a scale of 1 to 10 in his commitment to reaching them! I knew I had my work cut out for me in getting him to understand the importance of staying functional and active so he could enjoy his retirement years. We went to work on his posture, flexibility and balance. He comes to train with the 5:30 a.m. group and I love his workout ethic. He has been a part of our community for more than four years, has run a few 5K races, partakes in adventure travel, hunts, snowmobiles and enjoys his grandkids. Pat is an excellent role model for the aging population Here is what Pat has to say:

"I have been a member of the Westminster Fit Body community for a little over 4 years. I heard about the program when Lisa met with me about renting our building for her large group training business. At the time, I knew I was working too much and not taking the best care of myself. I was feeling unfit and was slowing down. We talked about my goals and came up with a plan. This was the first time I had actually worked with a personal trainer and really enjoyed it. The workouts are fun, engaging and challenging and the last time I went for a physical, my doctor told me that whatever I was doing was working well, and to keep it up, as it's the best thing for me.

Lisa has helped me realize that I need to stay active and functional so I can continue going on travel adventures like. hiking in Costa Rica, snowmobiling with my wife, (I did a 3000 mile trip thru Canada) and playing with my grandkids. They spend the summers with us in our cabin up north and I need to be able to keep up with them. I also enjoy hunting and need to stay fit in order to hike the rugged terrain in Colorado and other areas. I would recommend this program to anyone who would like to stay functional and independent for as long as possible. Call Lisa Dumont just as soon as you can! You'll be glad you did!" - **Pat (72)**

Meet Barb- Pat's better half;)

"I have been attending Fit Body for about 2 years but started working with Lisa a couple of years earlier than that when Lisa was a personal trainer at the nearby fitness center. When I initially joined the program, I wanted to reach and maintain my ideal weight, learn to eat healthily and follow a consistent exercise program to keep me strong and active as I age. Although I have been active for most of my life, I really enjoy the inspiration and motivation I get while training at WFBBC. The workouts are challenging and fun, and they support me in participating in many activities outside of training."

"A few years ago I injured my shoulder in a serious snow mobile accident. I was sidelined from group training, however Lisa took the time to work with me personally to strengthen my shoulder, increase my range of motion and get me back to my fitness routine. By attending Fit Body on a regular basis, I am still able to do all the things that I enjoy, such as travel, hike, snowmobile, play with my grandkids and be active in my garden/yard. I would say my future goal in fitness is to keep doing all I can to stay functional and fit so I can continue to participate in the VT area 5k runs and adventure travel. Last year I traveled through the Canadian Rockies, river rafting and hiking. I'm positive that being consistent with my fitness program helped me enjoy the trip immensely.

Some advice I can give: If you are struggling with your fitness journey, don't give up. There are many ways to keep going and maybe you just need to find someone to give you some special attention to get you started. The trainers at Fit Body are very knowledgeable and supportive. There are many levels of fitness in the group sessions so anyone can feel comfortable and succeed. They will also help you create a nutritional program individual to your needs. This is important to me." - **Barb (73)**

Couples Who Play Together Stay Together

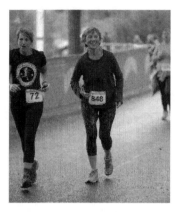

One of my favorite couples is the Dunbar's. Bev and Brad came in to my life many years ago and I'm happy to say are still with me. They are what I want to be when I grow up ☺. They have been married for thousands of years (I like to exaggerate!) and are passionate about keeping their bodies and minds healthy. I love that they are always open to participating in all the crazy ways I try to incorporate member incentive programs into my group. They continue to work not only on their personal growth at the young ages of 74 and 76, but realize that consistency in self-care is key to maintaining independence. Brad's posture and flexibility have improved immensely as we work on core strength and function. Bev's confidence in her body continues to grow as she maintains a beautiful, healthy body composition.

It's now time for them to tell you their side of the story:

BEV: "While participating in other exercise classes, I often questioned if I was using proper form and was worried about hurting myself. I thereby avoided many movements and didn't feel I was getting a good workout.

Because I felt comfortable with the trainers at WFBBC/FBF I knew I would get a good workout using their suggestions for exercise alternatives and their guidance on proper form that would support my individual goals and not cause undue discomfort. This gave me the confidence to progress in a healthy, safe way.

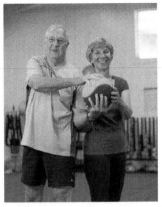

My initial goal was to stay active and improve my upper body strength. So many times in my daily life, I have the realization that if I was not training with WFBBC/FBF, I would have to rely on others to do things for me. My upper body strength is much better and I can spend time in my perennial garden pain-free now when in the past there were many months that I could not do so without experiencing discomfort.

I would urge anyone wanting to stay active to join Fit Body. I have had to get past the feeling of being too old and realize now that what we do in training flows into every aspect of my daily life."

BRAD: "I joined Fit Body with encouragement from my wife and the desire to improve my physical well-being. I enjoy the group sessions because it is not only rewarding to experience my personal progress but to see that of fellow campers. The enthusiasm and knowledge of the staff and their willingness to help every camper no matter what level they may be at or start at, is one thing that sets this program apart from the others out there. They sincerely care about us. "

My initial goals were to be stronger, have more energy and lose weight. I am experiencing success in all three areas while also learning better lifestyle choices. It is the best gift you can give yourself and those who love you."

Fitness Ambassador Extraordinaire

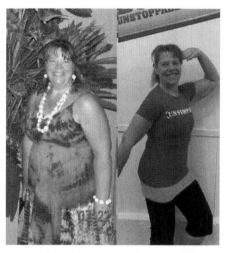

We met Pam more than 5 years ago when she was invited by her sister to support a 3 hour bootcamp – a - thon fundraiser called "Burn the Fat, Feed the Hungry." Little did she know that her initial intent of supporting a good cause would turn into learning about lifelong habits to support health and fitness. Over the past 5+ years she has transformed in so many ways. High blood pressure is no longer an issue, she is at a healthy body composition, having lost over 80 lbs. and she continues to focus on all aspects of her self-care at Fit Body. She is a star with her picture proudly displayed up on our Transformation Board.

Pam is enjoying her new-found strength, and her improved range of motion. She shows up regularly to the 5:30 am training despite having to travel quite a distance to get to Westminster Fit Body. She has made some close friends along the way and supports many of our new members by helping them feel comfortable and welcome. Way to go, Pam! You are an inspiration to all of us and a true Fitness Ambassador! - **Pam (56)**

Training for Hip Surgery and Beyond

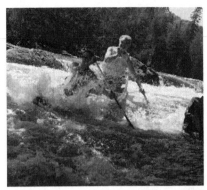 Guy came into Westminster Fit Body in April 2012. He has a quiet demeanor, a wealth of knowledge on all kinds of topics, a huge heart and a desire to continue to work on his self-care. His initial goal was to control his weight and have enough mobility in his hip to get his leg over his motorcycle easily and effortlessly! He has accomplished this and so much more! He lost over 40lbs, built up his body strength and mobility AND dramatically improved his overall balance. Guy never stops moving, even after going thru a full hip replacement and knee surgery. He continues to go on physical adventures, like climbing mountains, canoeing down raging rivers, and traveling the world every chance he gets both for pleasure and for humanitarian efforts. Did I mention he turned 70 this summer?

Here is what Guy had to say about boot camp when he initially came in to Fit Body:

"I probably have to have hip surgery in the near future. I want to be physically in shape for the surgery, and using the program is a way to regain my physical condition, as I move, hopefully, to a long period of active and consistent exercise in my life.

It's often a lot of fun, yet challenging. And it makes all the difference to me that there is a coach training safe and effective classes, instead of me trying to think what I should do for exercise today to support my goals." - **Guy (70)**

Redefining "Grandma"

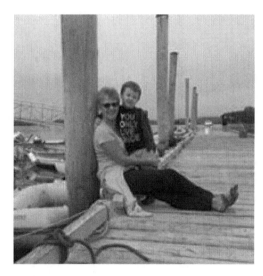

She breaks the mold of being a Grandma. Her name is Sue Higley - retired from a long time commitment to the US Postal Service, tall, beautiful inside and out, with beautiful silvery gray hair, and a good sport. She always comes in to train hard. It's hard to believe she's a grandmother!

Sue understands the importance of staying active, working out and eating right well into her retirement years and makes a great role model for my group. Her positive attitude always brings a special light to the trainings.

As a result of her training with us, she's doing 5k's with her kids, actively participating in the care of her grandchildren, and traveling, among many other things. When I asked her to say one thing about her participation at Westminster Fit Body, this is what she said: "The only thing I would add was that I NEVER considered myself athletic in ANY way. You have shown me there is SOME KIND of athlete in everyone. XO" - **Sue (57)**

Walking on the Wild Side!

Mary Lou has been attending the Fit Body program for just 2 months. She came to us because "she needed to ramp up her exercise routine, but wanted something that would help her to develop strength, flexibility, and stability safely without over-extending herself." She was an avid walker and walked 10,000 steps daily! "I have become almost obsessed with getting my 10,000 steps in every day, and not being satisfied with 6 or 7 thousand!" Walking supported her in maintaining her fitness level. However, she knew she needed to do more.

When she came through our doors, she was nervous to start because she did not want to over extend herself, yet she wanted to be challenged. Her physical education background made her knowledgeable of body mechanics, muscle function, and core strength but she never really utilized this knowledge until she heard "Tighten your core" so many times from the trainer that it has now become an automatic response to any type of movement she performs. Not only has she seen a change in strength, flexibility and stability, but she is also pleasantly surprised at the changes in her muscle tone and shape since participating in the workouts at Fit Body!

"My clothes fit better and I'm having FUN while making these changes! I have become very aware of how I move, particularly when I'm on unstable surfaces, reaching for things, or bending down. I am also very aware of automatically tightening my core muscles in all activities. I feel stronger and better about myself.

The trainers are very knowledgeable in the area of fitness for people in my age group. I am pleased with how each week, activities are changed, difficulty levels are increased, and how the Trainer individualizes instruction to meet the needs of each member of the class."

Her future fitness plans include continuing to use the concepts of Fit Body Forever, taking sessions, and building on what she has been practicing. She is so happy she worked up the courage to walk through Fit Body's doors and looks forward to enjoying her retirement years! - **Mary Lou (63)**

Team Sports again at 66!

"I'd been an athlete all my life, but I just couldn't make myself exercise consistently. In the past, I was always accountable to a team but I eventually lost the drive to stay consistent with my workouts even though I knew how important it is to stay active as we age. My partner had been participating in the Fit Body program for many years and tried repeatedly to get me to try it out. Well, I finally did and was pleasantly surprised at how fun the workouts were. The trainers are knowledgeable, supportive and always create challenging workouts to support strength, endurance, flexibility and balance using a variety of tools. Now, I feel "off" when I don't go workout. Everyone is so supportive and people take notice when I'm absent. This past summer, I was part of a team of women all ages, sizes and fitness levels who competed in the Mudderella - obstacle run. Two years ago, my partner and I spent three weeks riding our bikes through the rough terrain in Alaska. Training at Fit Body gave me the confidence again to compete in a team sport at 66 years young!" - **Becky (66)**

Health Is SO MUCH More Than Weight Loss

Corrie was reluctant to join Westminster Fit Body. She had done workout programs in the past and had not seen results fast enough so gave up. Two of her friends were trying out the program and talked her into coming along. She took advantage of a promotion that offered a short term trial to lose weight and make exercise a part of her life again.

Now the promotion is over, and Corrie is a full time member!!! Here is what she had to say:

"I love the support and overwhelming encouragement of the trainers. I love how I feel after a workout, especially a difficult one. I love that every day is different but always challenging. I love that when I am there it's all about me - no one else. It's my workout, I'm not compared to others and I'm not comparing myself to others (which, as a competitive person, is new for me). The nutritional guidance has also been very beneficial to me.

My initial goals were to lose weight and to find an exercise routine that would become a part of my day that I looked forward to doing (rather than dreading a workout or feeling like it was somethings HAD to do.) I have lost some weight and am confident that with the support of the TEAM at WFBBC, my ultimate weight goal will be achieved! I am excited that I have found a program that keeps me accountable and that I enjoy very much! It is my "ME" time" and I'm actually bummed when I don't make it for whatever reason.

Although at first I was worried about keeping up with everyone or being "good enough", I am so happy that I decided to try it out. The feeling you get when you finish a challenging workout is indescribable. WFFBC has been a game changer for both my physical and mental health and I am so grateful!! Just try it. You'll see what I mean." - **Corrie (37)**

Bringing A Ray of Sunshine to Every Training Session

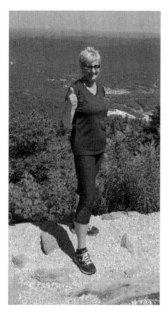

Sandy came in to Westminster Fit Body about 6 months ago. She had heard lots of good things about the program and finally decided to try it out. She is a ray of sunshine and always has a big smile on her face. She wants to stay fit and get stronger and feels that she is already experiencing success in both areas. Her golf game has improved and her new-found confidence in herself found her hiking to the top of Killington Mountain on her 63rd birthday this year. "I not only made it to the top, but I made it with no issues. Wow!" She also participated in a 5K run with the Forever Fit Team and looks forward to the race next year!

"I love bootcamp and the inspiration from all the wonderful coaches and campers. The workouts are challenging and fun and I love the way the coaches are willing to support every camper with modifications appropriate for their fitness level!" - **Sandy (63)**

Mudrunner Marsha

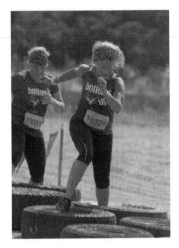

Marsha has been a member of Westminster Fit Body for several years. When she started, her attendance was not always consistent, until she had finally had enough, just before her 50th birthday.

Marsha stated; "I wanted to stop the cycle and just get stronger."

While her initial goal was to lose weight, she soon realized she really wanted to be stronger and have more endurance. And stronger she is, hiking the mountains (in the mud) of Ecuador, riding her motorcycle, chasing her 2-year-old grandson and just recently completing the Mudderella mud run and her first 5K. Marsha said, "I can say I do feel stronger. Three years ago I probably wouldn't have done half of these things. What I love about Fit Body is the encouragement and support you get from others. The Coaches are all great about finding ways to adjust the exercises to my ability. I love that every day is a new workout keeping it fresh. I've made many new friends to help keep me motivated and accountable to my program.

Everyone is there for the same thing: to live a healthy lifestyle and get stronger as we age. You don't have to be perfect at it, everyone has their own journey. Exercise does get addicting!" It's never too late to start." **- Marsha (50)**

It's Never Too Late to Find Your Inner-Athlete

"I have struggled with my weight most of my life and was a long-time Weight Watcher. One day, a co-worker asked me if I'd like to join her in a training session at Westminster Fit Body, a functional fitness program that had recently opened in our area. I thought at the time that I was just helping a friend stay accountable to her fitness program. Later I found out it was so much more. This friend soon found every excuse in the book not to continue. Not wanting to be a "quitter" I stayed on, and soon thereafter came to realize that the program was impacting me physically and emotionally like I hadn't experienced before. I remained a member of this caring community until the day I moved out of state to enjoy retirement. "

Never had I been considered an athlete. With the aid of the spring-loaded floor, Lisa's knowledge and purpose, fellow campers and staff, I discovered a true sense of accomplishment when I walked out of each workout."

My initial goal was to lose weight. While I have not as of yet achieved what I perceive to be my 'goal', with Lisa's counseling I have been able to better understand what is more important than the scale. We call them Non-scale victories!

What I did 'reach' was the confidence level that has allowed me to take part in several different physical activities on a daily basis. Weight loss is not a measure of health.

I have promoted Westminster's Fit Body program since the first session I attended. It is because of this experience that I chose to retire to a place that is considered "America's Most Active Retirement Community" so that I have an opportunity to remain physically active in many ways — there are hundreds of opportunities to engage in activity programs here."

Thank you Fit Body Team! - **Doreen** *(68)*

You've Got to Move it, Move it"

I'll never forgot the day he first walked thru my doors and stepped onto the red carpet of vulnerability. His name is Wayne- in his 70's an engineer, retired from owning a successful business and enjoying a life of travel, playing music, enjoying his grandkid, riding his motorcycle and staying active.

He so reminded me of my dad- tall, glasses, not easy to "read", quiet but with a dry sense of humor. I couldn't wait to see how his transformation would go. I could see that we definitely needed to work on his flexibility. We had a short and sweet conversation about his goals as I orientated him about the program and what to expect. Two years later, it's amazing to see how far he's come in all areas of fitness. It's now time for him to tell you his side of the story. and it wasn't easy:

Below is a series of questions we sent out to Wayne- as you can see he is a short and sweet kind of guy!

FBF: What compelled you to join FBBC? W: Shamed into it by daughter although I knew she was right - "... you got to move it, move it..."

FBF: What do you love about Westminster Fit Body? W: Love is too much. Tolerate is the operative word.

FBF: What were your initial goals? W: to survive every session and to keep coming 3 times a week. After a couple years my goal was to undertake Lisa's 60 day lose 20 lb. diet regimen and to my great surprise it worked - and now I love whole grains! I continue to drink HUGE quantities of lemon and cranberry flavored water, every day. And now I restrict red meat and food stuff that hasn't any real value.

FBF: Anything else you would like to tell others? W: I recommend FBBC to anybody who will listen. Even old guys like me. - **Wayne (72)**

Meet Tress and her New Sense of Confidence

"Every time I drove by Westminster Fit Body, I would say to myself," 'you need to stop in and check it out.' Plus, my friend was telling me that working out at Westminster Fit Body with Lisa was awesome. She told me how supportive Lisa was and how much better she felt. For a while, I was fearful of participating in the program because I am a bit competitive (figured I would hurt myself trying to keep up) and I had a chronic knee injury. This spring I saw an ad on Facebook for a 21 Day promotional workout program and something inside me said "just do it" so I did!" My knee was very painful and swollen at the time but working out on the spring loaded floor did not irritate it. In fact, my knee began to feel better the first week I attended. And I'm keeping up!

My goal was to increase my health and wellness. I knew from the minute I met Lisa, I was in the right place. Lisa went above and beyond my interest in health.

The trainings are not only safe and effective, but always bring a level of playfulness and fun. So many things have changed since I started 6 months ago. I've lost 10 pounds, my sleep is much better and I feel younger and lighter on my feet. I can't believe how good I feel. I'm more focused at my job and there are no more afternoon crashes. I feel more confident in my life, my body, in speaking my truth. A co-worker said I look like a different person, even wondering if I had a face lift. I feel like a different person- a happier, bouncier, playful, more confident person.

I love the community and plan on making this a lifelong commitment."

Thank you Lisa, Mark, Ann, Laura, Ronna, Bob, and Sarah! - **Tress (58)**

Can You Imagine It?

What might your testimonial be? What might your story 6 months or 6 years from now be if you take charge of your health and fitness…and more importantly your aging trajectory?

For just a moment I want you to ponder this…you have an age number in your head at which you expect your life will end. It is in there whether you admit it or not so close your eyes and focus on what age you think you will be when you die. Okay, got it?

Now add ten years to that number.

Now add 15 years to that number!

If you were to live 10 years or 15 years longer than you ever imagined, how might your life need to change this year or this month or this week…or even today?

Get Ready for Your
Best Years Yet

Hi, I'm Dr. Dan Ritchie, President and Co-Founder of the Functional Aging Institute. It's our passion to train and equip certified functional aging experts like Lisa Dumont and her team of coaches. Because they have made this additional investment in their expertise, your trainers are among the most elite authority experts in aging and fitness.

The question really sits with you now and what you make of all this. Can the unique design of functional exercises not only add years to your life, but enhance the quality of those years? What if you live to be 10 years older than you can even imagine? These are questions we really want you to think deeply about. We believe the research is very clear that the aging process can be positively impacted by the right kinds of exercise. The trajectory you are on for your functional ability in your 70s, 80s and 90s is directly related to the actions you are taking right now with respect to physical training to maintain your body.

It is tempting to think that we have nothing left to accomplish in the last 20 years of our life and that our "best" or most productive years will be behind us. If that is so, then why bother to put in all of this effort with an exercise program now? We want to share an inspiring story about a man you have probably all heard about whose biggest accomplishment came in his mid to late 70's. He was in prison for 27 years from the age of 45 (1962) to the age of 72 (1990). During those years he experienced horrible conditions, inadequate food, and most likely abusive treatment. But despite all of that he maintained a regular regime of pushups, sit-ups and running in place. There was a 3 year period where he was in a shared cell large enough to run small laps much to the annoyance of his fellow cell-mates. After being released from prison (at the age of 72) he rejoined the political movement he had started over 25 years earlier. Three years later, Nelson Mandela was elected president of South Africa and was eventually awarded the Nobel Peace Prize.

It is safe to conclude that his 27 year fitness regimen significantly contributed to his significance and success upon release. If Nelson Mandela had emerged from prison a frail, weak, broken "old" man he certainly would not have been able to become the inspirational leader for his country and the rest of the world that he is fondly remembered as being. We could either say that the most productive years of his life were taken from him or we could say that age is just a number…one that shouldn't hold us back from being the best that we can be.

What do you have yet to accomplish? A major achievement in your field? Amazing adventures? Dancing with your grand-daughter at her wedding? Expeditions. Vacations. Excursions. Adventures. Whatever your endeavor, we know you have a significant purpose or calling for every single one of your remaining years. We hope you make the investment in yourself to live those years with more gusto, energy, enthusiasm and joy than you ever thought possible.

Sincerely,

Dan M. Ritchie, PhD
Co-founder, Funtional Aging Institute

Lisa Dumont

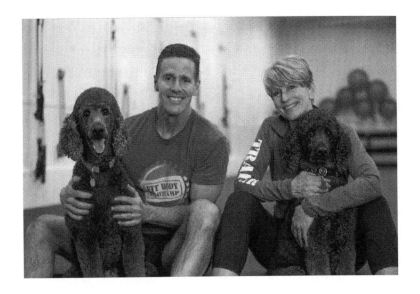

My Story

I've worked in the field of Health and Wellness since 1983, when I graduated from the University of Connecticut,

Storrs, with a Bachelor of Science Degree in Nutrition. The only reason (or so I thought at the time) I picked this major was because I, like many other freshmen gained...... the infamous "Freshman Ten"- 10 pounds that is! I was already a shy kid who lacked self-confidence so gaining weight only messed even more with my self-image, which resulted in an eating disorder. Turning lemons into lemonade, I seized the opportunity to break down my self-imposed limits and changed my major to Nutritional Sciences with the sole intention of beating the disorder. Little did I know at the time, but my degree would eventually play such a big part in my mission: Healthy People, Healthy Planet, LLC born in 2007!

Upon Graduation, I promptly moved to Southern California to "find myself" and continue my education at San Diego State University, studying exercise physiology. I worked for an amazing chiropractor as a chiropractic assistant and nutritionist, and was in charge of creating stretching programs. This is where I became very interested in keeping our bodies in balance structurally (personal training/chiropractic) as well as chemically (nutrition). I worked with many older patients, giving them gentle stretching and strengthening programs and saw positive results. Helping them move freely built their confidence. This was very rewarding and my first "aha" that drove my passion to help others live a healthy and full life.

Then, I turned 40. Everyone told me, "get ready.... You are going to gain a bunch of fat around your belly when you hit 40." I don't believe everything I hear, so I went on a mission to prove everyone wrong. I got a belly button ring to keep me focused and learned all I could about the body, hormones, women, weight training., etc. I was introduced to Metabolic Resistance training/functional training which led me to quick, effective workouts coupled with eating healthy. This became a huge part of my successful formula to maintain a healthy body composition for the next 10 years. Boy, did I prove them wrong!

Then, I turned 50. I had opened up a new studio barely a year earlier to train larger groups with my unstoppable fitness formula but was sidelined when I was told I had uterine cancer. My first question was, "How could this happen to me? I'm such a fake, Here I am, teaching everyone how to be healthy and take care of themselves and I got cancer!" My doctor assured me that it can happen to anyone.   Here is where Mia – my first standard poodle, came in to my life. I begged my husband for a puppy (little did he know I already had her picked out;) and had put a deposit down) and told him that if he let me get a puppy I would obey the doctor. and stay in bed to heal for three weeks. (The doctor initially said 6 weeks so we compromised.) I learned that I am not invincible, even if I'm certain my "healthy people healthy mission" came from above. Hence yet another opportunity to turn lemons into lemonade. I lay low for three weeks to heal my body, mind, and spirit with my "Here and Now puppy" Mia. Soon I was strong enough to get back to my mission........ supporting as many people as possible making their health a priority until it's my time to leave this planet.

Fast-forward 7 years: I'm still happily in the business of teaching my clients how to make their self-care a priority, training groups, educating, motivating, and CARING! Now that I'm 56, I can appreciate that as I continue to make choices on a daily basis to promote health and wellness, I WILL be able to do all those things I desire to do- travel, ride horseback, play with grandkids (hopefully someday!), give back to my community, be of service, hike, **AND most of all support all of you who are willing to overcome your fears and concerns about aging and exercise by focusing on your goals and dreams. The goal is to preserve your independence for as long as possible.**

What do you say, are you in? Read on and take advantage of my Special Offer at the back of the book to get started.

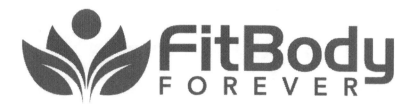

Westminster Fit Body/Fit Body Forever

www.westminsterfbf.com

5983 US RTE 5

WESTMINSTER, VT 05158

802.722.3460

www.facebook.com/westminsterfitbodyforever